KEGEL EXERCISE

Empower Your Pelvic Health In-Depth Techniques And Benefits Of Kegel Exercises For Everyone With Essential Kegel Exercise Routines For Optimal Health And Fitness

CONTENTS

1: Introduction

2: Understanding the Pelvic Floor

3: Benefits of Kegel Exercises

4: Getting Started with Kegel Exercises

5: Advanced Kegel Techniques

6: Kegel Exercises for Specific Populations

7: Combining Kegel Exercises with Other Practices

8: Conclusion

INTRODUCTION

Welcome to "Kegel Exercise," a comprehensive guide dedicated to enhancing your understanding and practice of Kegel exercises. This book aims to illuminate the profound benefits of Kegel exercises, providing you with the knowledge and tools necessary to improve your pelvic floor strength and overall well-being.

A. Purpose of the Book:

The primary objective of this book is to highlight the significance of Kegel exercises in promoting better health and well-being. These simple yet powerful exercises are designed to strengthen the pelvic floor muscles, which play a crucial role in various bodily functions. By engaging in regular Kegel exercises, individuals can experience improved bladder control, enhanced sexual health, and a reduction in the risk of pelvic organ prolapse. This book delves into the science behind these benefits, offering practical advice and step-by-step instructions to help you integrate Kegel exercises into your daily routine.

B. Benefits and Importance of Kegel Exercises:

Kegel exercises offer numerous health advantages, making them an essential practice for individuals of all ages and genders. Strengthening the pelvic floor can lead to better control over urinary and bowel movements, a crucial benefit for those dealing with incontinence. Additionally, these exercises can enhance sexual satisfaction by increasing muscle tone and blood flow to the pelvic region. For postpartum women, Kegel exercises can aid in recovery and help prevent complications related to childbirth. By understanding and practicing these exercises, you can significantly improve your quality of life and maintain your pelvic health.

Target Audience:

This book is tailored for individuals who are keen on improving their pelvic floor strength and health. Whether you are experiencing specific pelvic floor issues, such as incontinence or pelvic organ prolapse, or simply looking to enhance your overall well-being, this guide is for you. It is suitable for people of all fitness levels and ages, providing a valuable resource for those new to Kegel exercises as well as those seeking to deepen their practice.

C. Overview of Kegel Exercises:

Brief History and Origin:

Kegel exercises, named after Dr. Arnold Kegel, were first introduced in the late 1940s. Dr. Kegel, a gynecologist, developed these exercises as a non-surgical method to help women strengthen their pelvic floor muscles, primarily to treat urinary incontinence. Since their inception, Kegel exercises have gained widespread recognition for their effectiveness and have been adapted to benefit both men and women.

Basic Explanation of What Kegel Exercises Are:

Kegel exercises involve the repetitive contraction and relaxation of the pelvic floor muscles. These muscles support the bladder, bowel, and, in women, the uterus. The exercises can be performed anywhere and at any time, making them a convenient addition to your daily routine. To perform a Kegel exercise, you simply tighten your pelvic floor muscles as if you are trying to stop the flow of urine, hold the contraction for a few seconds, and then relax. Regular practice can lead to stronger pelvic muscles and improved control over pelvic functions.

UNDERSTANDING THE PELVIC FLOOR

A. Anatomy of the Pelvic Floor:

I. Detailed Description of the Pelvic Floor Muscles:

The pelvic floor is a complex and vital structure composed of a network of muscles, ligaments, and connective tissues that span the bottom of the pelvis. This hammock-like structure supports the pelvic organs, which include the bladder, intestines, and, in women, the uterus. Understanding the anatomy of the pelvic floor is crucial for recognizing its importance and the role it plays in overall health and bodily function.

1. Levator Ani Muscle Group:

adapted to benefit both men and women.

Basic Explanation of What Kegel Exercises Are:

Kegel exercises involve the repetitive contraction and relaxation of the pelvic floor muscles. These muscles support the bladder, bowel, and, in women, the uterus. The exercises can be performed anywhere and at any time, making them a convenient addition to your daily routine. To perform a Kegel exercise, you simply tighten your pelvic floor muscles as if you are trying to stop the flow of urine, hold the contraction for a few seconds, and then relax. Regular practice can lead to stronger pelvic muscles and improved control over pelvic functions.

UNDERSTANDING THE PELVIC FLOOR

A. Anatomy of the Pelvic Floor:

I. Detailed Description of the Pelvic Floor Muscles:

The pelvic floor is a complex and vital structure composed of a network of muscles, ligaments, and connective tissues that span the bottom of the pelvis. This hammock-like structure supports the pelvic organs, which include the bladder, intestines, and, in women, the uterus. Understanding the anatomy of the pelvic floor is crucial for recognizing its importance and the role it plays in overall health and bodily function.

1. Levator Ani Muscle Group:

Pubococcygeus (PC) Muscle: This muscle extends from the pubic bone to the coccyx (tailbone) and surrounds the openings of the urethra, vagina (in women), and anus. It plays a key role in maintaining continence and supports pelvic organs.

Iliococcygeus Muscle: Positioned laterally to the pubococcygeus, it also extends from the pelvic bones to the coccyx, providing additional support to the pelvic organs and contributing to the elevation of the anus.

Puborectalis Muscle: This U-shaped muscle wraps around the rectum, creating a sling that helps maintain fecal continence by keeping the anorectal angle intact.

2. Coccygeus Muscle:

Located posteriorly, this muscle extends from the ischial spine to the coccyx and sacrum, providing support to the pelvic floor and assisting with the stabilization of the sacroiliac joint.

3. Urogenital Diaphragm:

This layer of muscles, including the deep transverse perineal muscle, stretches across the anterior part of the pelvic outlet. It supports the pelvic organs and plays a role in urinary continence.

4. Perineal Body:

This fibromuscular structure lies between the vaginal opening and the anus in women, and between the scrotum and the anus in men. It serves as an anchor point for several pelvic floor muscles and is crucial for the integrity of the pelvic floor.

II. Functions of the Pelvic Floor:

The pelvic floor muscles perform several essential functions that are vital for maintaining health and well-being:

1. Supportive Function: The pelvic floor provides critical support for the pelvic organs, preventing prolapse. This is especially important during activities that increase intra-abdominal pressure, such as lifting, coughing, or straining.

2. Continence: The pelvic floor muscles are key players in maintaining both urinary and fecal

continence. They contract to close the urethra and anus, preventing involuntary leakage, and relax to allow for controlled urination and defecation.

3. Sexual Function: In women, the pelvic floor muscles contribute to sexual arousal and orgasm by increasing vaginal tightness and enhancing sensation. In men, these muscles support erectile function and ejaculation.

4. Stabilization: The pelvic floor muscles work in conjunction with the core muscles, including the diaphragm, abdominal muscles, and back muscles, to stabilize the pelvis and spine, promoting good posture and reducing the risk of injury.

B. Common Pelvic Floor Issues:

I. Causes and Symptoms of Pelvic Floor Dysfunction:

Pelvic floor dysfunction occurs when the pelvic floor muscles are weakened, overly tight, or otherwise impaired, leading to a range of symptoms and complications. Understanding the causes and recognizing the symptoms is crucial for early intervention and effective treatment.

1. Causes of Pelvic Floor Dysfunction:

Childbirth: Vaginal delivery can stretch and weaken the pelvic floor muscles, especially if there is prolonged pushing or the use of forceps.

Aging: The natural aging process leads to a loss of muscle tone and elasticity in the pelvic floor.

Surgery: Pelvic surgeries, such as hysterectomy, can damage or weaken pelvic floor muscles.

Obesity: Excess weight increases pressure on the pelvic floor, leading to muscle strain and weakening.

Chronic Coughing: Conditions like chronic bronchitis or asthma can lead to repeated stress on the pelvic floor muscles.

Heavy Lifting: Repeated heavy lifting or high-impact activities can strain and weaken the pelvic floor.

2. Symptoms of Pelvic Floor Dysfunction:

Urinary Incontinence: This includes stress incontinence (leakage during activities like coughing or laughing) and urge incontinence (a sudden, intense urge to urinate).

Fecal Incontinence: Inability to control bowel movements, leading to unintentional leakage.

Pelvic Organ Prolapse: A sensation of heaviness or pressure in the pelvic area, often described as a feeling that something is falling out of the vagina.

Pelvic Pain: Chronic pain in the pelvic region, which may be associated with intercourse, urination, or bowel movements.

Sexual Dysfunction: Pain during intercourse (dyspareunia), reduced sensation, or difficulty achieving orgasm.

II. Impact on Quality of Life:

Pelvic floor dysfunction can significantly affect an individual's quality of life, impacting physical, emotional, and social well-being.

1. Physical Impact:

Reduced Mobility: Pain and discomfort can limit physical activity, leading to decreased mobility and fitness.

Chronic Discomfort: Persistent pain and discomfort in the pelvic region can affect daily activities and overall physical health.

2. Emotional Impact:

Stress and Anxiety: Concerns about incontinence and pelvic pain can lead to heightened stress and anxiety.

Depression: The chronic nature of pelvic floor issues and their impact on daily life can contribute to feelings of depression and hopelessness.

3. Social Impact:

Isolation: Fear of incontinence accidents or pain can lead to social withdrawal and isolation.

Impact on Relationships: Sexual dysfunction and chronic pain can strain intimate relationships, reducing overall quality of life.

THE BENEFITS OF KEGEL EXERCISES

A. Health Benefits:

Kegel exercises, also known as pelvic floor exercises, offer a multitude of health benefits that can significantly improve one's quality of life. This chapter will delve into the various advantages of incorporating Kegel exercises into your daily routine, focusing on improved bladder and bowel control, enhanced sexual health, and postpartum recovery.

I. Improved Bladder and Bowel Control:

One of the most significant health benefits of Kegel exercises is the improvement in bladder and bowel control. These exercises strengthen the pelvic floor muscles, which support the bladder, bowel, and uterus. When these muscles are weak, issues such as urinary incontinence and fecal incontinence can arise.

1. Urinary Incontinence: Strengthening the pelvic floor muscles can help prevent and manage urinary incontinence. This condition, characterized by the involuntary leakage of urine, is common among women, especially those who have given birth, undergone menopause, or are aging. Men can also benefit from Kegel exercises, particularly after prostate surgery. Regular Kegel exercises can reduce the frequency and severity of leaks, providing greater control over the bladder.

2. Fecal Incontinence: Similarly, Kegel exercises can help manage fecal incontinence, the inability to control bowel movements. By strengthening the muscles that support the rectum, individuals can experience better control and fewer incidents of accidental bowel leakage.

II. Enhanced Sexual Health:

Kegel exercises are also renowned for their positive impact on sexual health. By strengthening the pelvic floor muscles, individuals can experience more satisfying sexual experiences and improved overall sexual function.

1. For Women: Strong pelvic floor muscles can lead to increased sensitivity and stronger orgasms.

Women who regularly perform Kegel exercises often report greater sexual pleasure and satisfaction. These exercises can also help manage conditions like vaginismus, where involuntary muscle spasms can make intercourse painful.

2. For Men: Men can benefit from Kegel exercises through improved erectile function and greater control over ejaculation. Strengthened pelvic floor muscles can help in achieving and maintaining erections, as well as in prolonging the duration of sexual activity.

III. Postpartum Recovery:

The postpartum period can be challenging for new mothers, as the body undergoes significant changes and recovery processes. Kegel exercises can play a crucial role in this recovery, helping new mothers regain strength and functionality in their pelvic floor muscles.

1. Strengthening Muscles: During childbirth, the pelvic floor muscles can become stretched and weakened. Performing Kegel exercises can help new mothers strengthen these muscles, reducing the risk of urinary incontinence and pelvic organ prolapse.

2. Promoting Healing: Kegel exercises increase blood flow to the pelvic region, promoting

healing and reducing the risk of infections. This can be particularly beneficial for women who have experienced perineal tears or episiotomies during delivery.

B. Psychological Benefits:

In addition to the physical health benefits, Kegel exercises offer a range of psychological benefits that can enhance overall well-being. These exercises can increase body awareness, boost confidence, and improve self-esteem.

I. Increased Body Awareness:

Engaging in Kegel exercises requires a heightened awareness of the pelvic floor muscles and their function. This increased body awareness can lead to a deeper connection with one's physical self and a better understanding of bodily functions.

1. Mind-Body Connection: By focusing on the pelvic floor muscles during exercises, individuals can develop a stronger mind-body connection. This can enhance overall mindfulness and awareness, leading to improved mental health and well-being.

2. Body Control: Improved awareness and control over the pelvic floor muscles can translate into better overall body control. This can enhance coordination and balance, contributing to better physical performance in various activities.

II. Boosted Confidence and Self-Esteem:

The psychological benefits of Kegel exercises extend to boosting confidence and self-esteem. Feeling in control of one's body and experiencing improvements in physical health can have a profound impact on mental and emotional well-being.

1. Empowerment: Mastering Kegel exercises and experiencing their benefits can create a sense of empowerment. Individuals may feel more capable and in control of their health, leading to increased confidence.

2. Improved Sexual Confidence: Enhanced sexual health resulting from Kegel exercises can also

boost sexual confidence. Feeling more in tune with one's body and experiencing greater sexual satisfaction can lead to improved self-esteem and a more positive self-image.

Kegel exercises offer a wide array of benefits that extend beyond just physical health. By improving bladder and bowel control, enhancing sexual health, aiding in postpartum recovery, increasing body awareness, and boosting confidence and self-esteem, these exercises can significantly enhance one's overall quality of life. Incorporating Kegel exercises into your daily routine can lead to a healthier, more confident, and more empowered you.

GETTING STARTED WITH KEGEL EXERCISES

Embarking on the journey of Kegel exercises can be both empowering and transformative. By strengthening your pelvic floor muscles, you can improve bladder control, enhance sexual health, and support overall pelvic health. This chapter will guide you through the initial steps of identifying the right muscles, mastering basic Kegel techniques, and establishing a consistent routine.

A. Identifying the Right Muscles:

Before you can effectively perform Kegel exercises, it is crucial to identify and engage the correct muscles – the pelvic floor muscles. These muscles support the bladder, bowel, and, for women, the uterus.

I. Techniques to Locate and Engage Pelvic Floor Muscles

1. Stopping Urine Midstream:

One of the simplest ways to locate your pelvic floor muscles is to try stopping your urine flow midstream. If you can do this, you have successfully engaged the correct muscles. However, avoid making this a habit as it can lead to incomplete emptying of the bladder and increase the risk of urinary tract infections.

2. Visualizing the Muscles:

Imagine you are trying to hold in gas or prevent yourself from passing wind. The muscles you use to do this are your pelvic floor muscles.

3. Using a Mirror:

For women, using a mirror can help you see the muscles in action. Insert a finger into your vagina and try to squeeze and lift around it. You should feel a tightening around your finger.

4. Consulting a Professional:

If you are unsure whether you are engaging the right muscles, consider consulting a healthcare provider, such as a pelvic floor therapist. They can provide guidance and ensure you are performing the exercises correctly.

B. Basic Kegel Techniques:

Once you have identified your pelvic floor muscles, you can begin practicing basic Kegel techniques. These exercises are straightforward but require focus and consistency.

I. Step-by-Step Guide to Performing Kegel Exercises:

1. Find a Comfortable Position:

Start by lying down or sitting in a comfortable position. As you become more proficient, you can perform Kegels in any position.

2. Engage Your Pelvic Floor Muscles:

Tighten your pelvic floor muscles and hold the contraction for a count of three to five seconds. Ensure you are not contracting your abdominal, thigh, or buttock muscles.

3. Release and Relax:

Slowly release the contraction and relax your muscles completely for an equal count of three to five seconds.

4. Repeat the Exercise:

Aim to repeat the exercise 10 to 15 times per session. Perform three sessions daily: morning, afternoon, and evening.

II. Common Mistakes to Avoid:

1. Using the Wrong Muscles:

Ensure you are engaging only your pelvic floor muscles. Avoid tightening your abdomen, thighs, or buttocks.

2. Holding Your Breath:

Breathe normally throughout the exercise. Holding your breath can add unnecessary pressure to your abdomen and pelvic floor.

3. Overdoing It:

Avoid over-exercising. Excessive Kegel exercises can lead to muscle fatigue and even weaken the pelvic floor.

4. Neglecting Relaxation:

Ensure you fully relax your muscles between contractions.

Constantly keeping your muscles tense can lead to muscle strain.

C. Frequency and Routine:

Establishing a regular routine is vital for the effectiveness of Kegel exercises. Consistency will lead to stronger and more resilient pelvic floor muscles.

I. Recommended Daily Routines:

1. Start Small:

Begin with three sets of 10 repetitions daily. As your muscles become stronger, you can gradually increase the duration of each contraction and the number of repetitions.

2. Incorporate into Daily Activities:

Integrate Kegels into your daily routine. Perform them while brushing your teeth, watching TV, or waiting at a traffic light.

3. Track Your Progress:

Keep a journal to monitor your progress. Note the duration and number of repetitions to see how you improve over time.

II. Tips for Consistency and Progression:

1. Set Reminders:

Use alarms or phone reminders to ensure you remember to perform your exercises regularly.

2. Stay Patient:

Pelvic floor strengthening takes time. Be patient and stay consistent, as results may take a few weeks to become noticeable.

3. Gradually Increase Difficulty:

As your muscles strengthen, increase the duration of each contraction up to 10 seconds and add more repetitions per set.

4. Incorporate Advanced Techniques:

Once you master basic Kegels, you can explore advanced techniques like quick flicks (rapid contractions and releases) or holding contractions for longer periods.

ADVANCED KEGEL TECHNIQUES

A. Progressive Training:

As you progress in your Kegel exercise regimen, it's essential to gradually increase the intensity and duration of your workouts. This progressive approach ensures that your pelvic floor muscles continue to strengthen and become more resilient over time. In this section, we will delve into strategies for intensifying your Kegel exercises and adding resistance to your routine.

I. Increasing Intensity and Duration:

To enhance the effectiveness of your Kegel exercises, start by gradually increasing both the intensity and duration of each session. Here are some guidelines to help you progress:

1. Start Slow and Steady: If you're new to Kegels, begin with basic contractions. Hold each contraction for about three seconds, then release for three seconds. Repeat this ten times. As you become more comfortable, gradually extend the hold time to five, then ten seconds.

2. Increase Repetitions: Once you can comfortably hold each contraction for ten seconds, start increasing the number of repetitions. Aim to complete three sets of ten contractions, three times a day.

3. Vary the Intensity: Introduce variations in the intensity of your contractions. Perform a set of quick, strong squeezes followed by slower, more sustained contractions. This variation will challenge your muscles in different ways, promoting overall strength.

4. Practice Consistently: Consistency is key. Aim to practice Kegels daily, gradually building up to more extended and intense sessions over several weeks.

II. Adding Resistance:

Adding resistance to your Kegel exercises can further enhance muscle strength and endurance. Here are some effective methods to introduce resistance into your routine:

1. Use Kegel Weights: Kegel weights, also known as vaginal weights or cones, are specially designed devices that you can insert into the vagina to provide resistance during exercises. Start with a lighter weight and gradually move to heavier ones as your muscles become stronger.

2. Incorporate a Kegel Exerciser: Kegel exercisers, like pelvic floor trainers, often come with biofeedback and resistance features. These devices can help you monitor your progress and ensure you're performing exercises correctly.

3. Engage in Functional Exercises: Combine Kegels with other physical activities. For instance, perform Kegels while doing squats

or bridges. This not only adds resistance but also integrates your pelvic floor muscles into more dynamic movements.

4. Partner-Assisted Kegels: If comfortable, you can engage in partner-assisted Kegels. During intercourse, try to squeeze your pelvic floor muscles around your partner's finger or a suitable object. This can add a different type of resistance and help you gain better control.

B. Incorporating Kegels into Daily Activities:

Integrating Kegel exercises into your daily routine can be highly effective, ensuring that you practice consistently without needing to set aside dedicated time. Here are some practical ways to incorporate Kegels into various activities throughout your day.

I. Exercises to Do While Sitting, Standing, and Lying Down:

1. While Sitting:

At Your Desk: Whether you're working or studying, take a few minutes every hour to perform a set of Kegels. Sit up straight, engage your pelvic floor muscles, hold for a few seconds, then release.

Watching TV: During commercial breaks or slow scenes, do a few sets of Kegels. This can make use of otherwise idle time.

2. While Standing:

Waiting in Line: Whether at the grocery store or the bank, standing in line provides an excellent opportunity to practice Kegels. Squeeze and release your pelvic floor muscles discreetly.

During Household Chores: Incorporate Kegels while doing activities like washing dishes or folding laundry. The key is to find moments when you can multitask.

3. While Lying Down:

Before Sleep: Incorporate a set of Kegels into your nightly routine. Lying down helps you isolate the pelvic floor muscles without engaging other muscle groups.

Upon Waking: Start your day with a few sets of Kegels before getting out of bed. This can be a gentle way to wake up your body and mind.

II. Practical Tips for Integration into Daily Life:

1. Set Reminders: Use your phone or a reminder app to alert you to perform Kegels at various times throughout the day. This can help build a consistent habit.

2. Link to Existing Habits: Pair Kegels with activities you already do regularly. For example, do a set every time you check your email or take a bathroom break.

3. Practice Mindfulness: Be mindful of your pelvic floor throughout the day. If you notice

you're clenching these muscles out of stress or habit, consciously relax them. Conversely, remind yourself to engage them during specific activities.

4. Stay Comfortable: Ensure you're comfortable and in a good posture when performing Kegels. Whether sitting, standing, or lying down, good posture supports proper muscle engagement.

5. Track Your Progress: Keep a journal or use an app to track your Kegel exercises. Note the duration, intensity, and any improvements you notice. This can help you stay motivated and see your progress over time.

KEGEL EXERCISES FOR SPECIFIC POPULATIONS

A. Women:

I. Prenatal and Postnatal Exercises:

Pregnancy and childbirth bring significant changes to a woman's body, particularly affecting the pelvic floor muscles. Kegel exercises can be a valuable tool for both prenatal and postnatal health.

Prenatal Kegel Exercises:

During pregnancy, the growing baby places increased pressure on the pelvic floor muscles. Strengthening these muscles can help support the uterus, bladder, and bowels, reducing the risk of incontinence and other complications.

1. Preparing for Childbirth: Regular Kegel exercises during pregnancy can improve muscle control, potentially making labor and delivery easier.

Strong pelvic floor muscles can help women push more effectively during labor, reducing the risk of prolonged labor and associated complications.

2. Preventing Incontinence:

Hormonal changes during pregnancy can weaken the pelvic floor muscles, leading to urinary incontinence.

Performing Kegel exercises can help maintain muscle strength and control, reducing the incidence of leakage.

Postnatal Kegel Exercises:

After childbirth, the pelvic floor muscles can be stretched and weakened, leading to various issues such as incontinence and pelvic organ prolapse.

1. Recovery and Healing:

Kegel exercises can aid in the recovery process by strengthening the pelvic floor muscles, helping them return to their pre-pregnancy state.

Gentle Kegel exercises can be started soon after childbirth, gradually increasing intensity as the muscles heal.

2. Preventing Long-term Complications:

Consistent postnatal Kegel exercises can help prevent long-term issues such as incontinence and pelvic organ prolapse, which can arise from weakened pelvic floor muscles.

II. Addressing Menopausal Changes:

Menopause brings a host of changes to a woman's body, many of which can affect the pelvic floor muscles. Hormonal fluctuations, particularly the decrease in estrogen, can lead to a weakening of these muscles.

Benefits of Kegel Exercises during Menopause:

1. Managing Incontinence:

Many women experience urinary incontinence during menopause due to the weakening of the pelvic floor muscles.

Regular Kegel exercises can help maintain muscle strength and control, reducing the incidence of leakage.

2. Supporting Pelvic Organs:

As estrogen levels decrease, the risk of pelvic organ prolapse increases.

Strengthening the pelvic floor muscles through Kegel exercises can provide better support for the bladder, uterus, and rectum, reducing the risk of prolapse.

3. Enhancing Sexual Health:

Menopausal changes can lead to a decrease in vaginal elasticity and lubrication, affecting sexual health and comfort.

Kegel exercises can increase blood flow to the pelvic region, improving muscle tone and potentially enhancing sexual pleasure and comfort.

B. Men:

I. Benefits for Prostate Health:

Kegel exercises are not just for women; they can also offer significant benefits for men's health, particularly in relation to prostate health.

Prostate Health Benefits:

1. Preventing Prostatitis:

Prostatitis, or inflammation of the prostate gland, can cause pain and urinary issues.

Regular Kegel exercises can improve pelvic floor muscle strength and support the prostate gland, potentially reducing the risk of prostatitis.

2. Post-Prostate Surgery Recovery:

Men who undergo prostate surgery, such as a prostatectomy, often experience urinary incontinence as a side effect.

Kegel exercises can help men regain bladder control by strengthening the pelvic floor muscles during recovery.

II. Improving Sexual Performance:

Kegel exercises can also play a role in enhancing men's sexual health and performance.

Sexual Health Benefits:

1. Improving Erectile Function:

Strong pelvic floor muscles can help improve blood flow to the penis, supporting erectile function.

Regular Kegel exercises can contribute to stronger and longer-lasting erections.

2. Enhancing Ejaculatory Control:

Kegel exercises can help men gain better control over their pelvic floor muscles, potentially improving ejaculatory control and reducing the risk of premature ejaculation.

3. Increasing Sexual Pleasure:

Strengthening the pelvic floor muscles can enhance overall muscle tone and control, potentially leading to increased sexual pleasure for both partners.

C. Elderly:

I. Maintaining Pelvic Floor Health with Age:

As individuals age, maintaining pelvic floor health becomes

increasingly important to prevent issues such as incontinence and pelvic organ prolapse.

Benefits of Kegel Exercises for the Elderly:

1. Preventing Incontinence:

Age-related muscle weakening can lead to urinary and fecal incontinence.

Regular Kegel exercises can help maintain muscle strength and control, reducing the risk of leakage.

2. Supporting Pelvic Organs:

With age, the risk of pelvic organ prolapse increases due to weakened pelvic floor muscles.

Strengthening these muscles through Kegel exercises can provide better support for pelvic organs, reducing the risk of prolapse.

II. Modifications for Physical Limitations:

For elderly individuals, it is important to modify Kegel exercises to accommodate physical limitations and ensure safety.

Modified Kegel Exercises:

1. Seated Kegel Exercises:

For those with limited mobility, seated Kegel exercises can be an effective alternative to traditional exercises performed while standing or lying down.

This modification allows individuals to perform exercises comfortably and safely.

2. Using Props and Supports:

Props such as exercise balls or cushions can provide additional support and stability during Kegel exercises.

This can help elderly individuals maintain proper form and reduce the risk of injury.

3. Gentle Progression:

It is important for elderly individuals to start with gentle exercises and gradually increase intensity as their muscle strength improves.

Consistent practice and gradual progression can help achieve the desired benefits without overexertion.

By understanding the specific needs and benefits of Kegel exercises for different populations, individuals can tailor their routines to achieve optimal pelvic floor health. Whether for prenatal and postnatal care, addressing menopausal changes, improving prostate health, enhancing sexual performance, or maintaining pelvic floor health with age, Kegel exercises offer a versatile and effective solution.

COMBINING KEGEL EXERCISES WITH OTHER PRACTICES

Integrating Kegel exercises into a comprehensive fitness and wellness routine can significantly enhance their effectiveness. This chapter explores how combining Kegel exercises with complementary exercises, a balanced diet, and stress management techniques can optimize pelvic floor health and overall well-being.

A. Complementary Exercises:

I. Yoga and Pilates for Pelvic Floor Strength:

Yoga and Pilates are excellent complements to Kegel exercises, as they both emphasize core strength, flexibility, and mindfulness. Specific poses and movements in these practices target the pelvic floor muscles, helping to reinforce the benefits of Kegels.

Yoga for Pelvic Floor Strength:

Certain yoga poses, such as the Bridge Pose (Setu Bandhasana), Child's Pose (Balasana), and Cat-Cow Pose (Marjaryasana-Bitilasana), directly engage the pelvic floor. These poses, when practiced regularly, can increase awarcness and control of these muscles.

Bridge Pose (Setu Bandhasana): This pose strengthens the glutes, lower back, and pelvic floor. By lifting the hips and engaging the core, practitioners can enhance the connection to their pelvic floor muscles.

Child's Pose (Balasana): A restorative pose that gently stretches the lower back and opens the hips, encouraging relaxation and blood flow to the pelvic region.

Cat-Cow Pose (Marjaryasana-Bitilasana): This dynamic movement sequence helps to mobilize the spine and pelvis, promoting flexibility and pelvic floor engagement.

Pilates for Pelvic Floor Strength:

Pilates focuses on core stability and strength, which includes the pelvic floor as a crucial component of the core muscle group.

Exercises like the Pelvic Curl, Hundred, and Spine Stretch Forward integrate pelvic floor activation.

Pelvic Curl: Similar to the Bridge Pose in yoga, this movement emphasizes rolling the spine off the mat and engaging the pelvic floor and core muscles.

Hundred: A challenging core exercise that requires deep abdominal engagement, indirectly strengthening the pelvic floor.

Spine Stretch Forward: This stretch promotes flexibility and encourages lengthening of the spine while maintaining pelvic floor activation.

II. Aerobic and Strength Training Compatibility:

Combining Kegel exercises with aerobic and strength training can provide a well-rounded fitness routine that supports overall pelvic health. Aerobic activities like walking, running, and swimming improve cardiovascular health, while strength training builds muscle and enhances body function.

Aerobic Exercise:

Regular aerobic exercise increases blood flow and improves overall health, which can positively affect pelvic floor function. Activities like brisk walking, cycling, and swimming are gentle on the pelvic floor while promoting cardiovascular fitness.

Brisk Walking: Enhances cardiovascular health and overall endurance without placing excessive strain on the pelvic floor.

Cycling: Low-impact aerobic exercise that strengthens the legs and core, indirectly supporting pelvic floor muscles.

Swimming: Provides a full-body workout that is gentle on the joints and pelvic floor, making it an excellent option for those with pelvic floor issues.

Strength Training:

Incorporating strength training exercises can further support pelvic floor health by improving muscle tone and coordination. Focus on exercises that engage the core and lower body while maintaining proper form to avoid undue stress on the pelvic floor.

Squats: A fundamental movement that strengthens the lower body and core. Ensure proper form to avoid excessive pressure on the pelvic floor.

Deadlifts: Engage the glutes, hamstrings, and lower back while promoting core stability. Proper technique is crucial to prevent pelvic floor strain.

Lunges: Improve balance and strength in the legs and core. Maintain pelvic floor engagement throughout the movement.

B. Holistic Approach to Pelvic Health:

A holistic approach to pelvic health involves not only physical exercises but also attention to diet, nutrition, and stress management. These factors play a crucial role in maintaining a healthy pelvic floor and overall well-being.

I. Diet and Nutrition:

A balanced diet rich in nutrients supports muscle function and overall health. Specific nutrients are essential for maintaining strong and healthy pelvic floor muscles.

Hydration: Adequate fluid intake is vital for muscle function and prevents urinary issues. Aim for at least 8 glasses of water per day.

Fiber: A diet high in fiber helps prevent constipation, reducing strain on the pelvic floor. Include plenty of fruits, vegetables, whole grains, and legumes.

Protein: Essential for muscle repair and growth. Include lean meats, dairy, beans, and nuts in your diet.

Magnesium: Supports muscle relaxation and function. Found in leafy greens, nuts, seeds, and whole grains.

II. Stress Management Techniques:

Chronic stress can negatively impact pelvic floor health by causing muscle tension and exacerbating issues like urinary incontinence. Incorporating stress management techniques can help maintain a healthy pelvic floor.

Mindfulness and Meditation:

Practicing mindfulness and meditation can reduce stress and promote relaxation, benefiting pelvic floor health. Techniques such as deep breathing, progressive muscle relaxation, and guided imagery can be particularly effective.

Deep Breathing: Encourages relaxation of the pelvic floor and reduces overall stress levels.

Progressive Muscle Relaxation: Involves tensing and relaxing different muscle groups, including the pelvic floor, to promote awareness and relaxation.

Guided Imagery: Uses visualization techniques to reduce stress and promote a sense of calm.

Lifestyle Modifications:

In addition to mindfulness practices, making lifestyle changes can help manage stress and improve pelvic floor health.

Regular Exercise: Physical activity is a natural stress reliever and can improve overall mood and well-being.

Adequate Sleep: Ensure you get enough restorative sleep to support overall health and reduce stress.

Healthy Work-Life Balance: Strive for a balance between work and personal life to minimize stress and promote well-being.

CONCLUSION

A. Summary of Key Points:

In this book, we have explored the profound benefits and techniques associated with Kegel exercises. These exercises, designed to strengthen the pelvic floor muscles, offer a range of health benefits for individuals of all genders. From improved bladder control and sexual health to enhanced core stability and postpartum recovery, the positive impacts of regular Kegel practice are extensive.

We began by understanding the anatomy and function of the pelvic floor muscles, laying the groundwork for appreciating the significance of these exercises. Following this foundational knowledge, we delved into the step-by-step techniques for performing Kegels correctly. Emphasis was placed on locating the pelvic floor muscles, ensuring proper form, and incorporating breathing techniques to maximize effectiveness. Variations and progressions of the basic Kegel were also covered, allowing practitioners to tailor their routines to their specific needs and fitness levels.

Furthermore, we discussed the common challenges and misconceptions associated with Kegel exercises, providing practical solutions and clarifications. The importance of consistency, patience, and proper technique was reiterated throughout, ensuring that readers are equipped with the knowledge and tools to practice safely and effectively.

B. Encouragement for Continued Practice:

Embarking on the journey of Kegel exercises is a commendable step towards improving your overall health and well-being. However, the true benefits are reaped through sustained, long-term practice. To maintain motivation and consistency, consider the following tips:

1. Set Realistic Goals: Establish achievable milestones and celebrate your progress, no matter how small. Tracking

improvements can boost your confidence and commitment.

2. Create a Routine: Integrate Kegel exercises into your daily schedule. Whether it's during morning routines, work breaks, or before bedtime, consistency is key.

3. Stay Informe: Keep learning about the benefits and variations of Kegel exercises. Understanding the evolving science and techniques can keep your practice fresh and engaging.

4. Join a Support Group: Connect with others who are also practicing Kegel exercises. Sharing experiences and challenges can provide mutual encouragement and accountability.

5. Listen to Your Body: Pay attention to how your body responds to the exercises. Adjust intensity and frequency as needed to avoid strain and ensure continued progress.

Remember, the journey of Kegel exercises is a marathon, not a sprint. Embrace the process and acknowledge the positive changes, both subtle and significant, that regular practice brings to your life.

C. Resources for Further Information:

To deepen your understanding and enhance your practice, consider exploring the following resources:

1. Recommended Reading:

Pelvic Power: Mind/Body Exercises for Strength, Flexibility, Posture, and Balance for Men and Women by Eric N. Franklin.

The Pelvic Floor Bible: Everything You Need to Know to Prevent and Cure Problems at Every Stage in Your Life by Jane Simpson.

Kegel Exercises For Men: Everything You Need to Know About Kegel Exercises for Men by Brian Smith.

2. Professional Guidance:

Pelvic Floor Physiotherapists: Seek advice from certified pelvic floor physiotherapists who can provide personalized assessments and tailored exercise plans.

Online Courses and Workshops: Participate in online courses and workshops led by experts in pelvic health and fitness.

Healthcare Providers: Consult your healthcare provider for recommendations on integrating Kegel exercises into your overall health regimen.

By utilizing these resources, you can continue to build on the foundation established in this book, ensuring a comprehensive and informed approach to your Kegel exercise practice.

Kegel exercises are a powerful tool for enhancing pelvic floor strength and overall well-being. Through understanding the techniques, staying motivated, and seeking further information, you can sustain a lifelong practice that yields significant health benefits. Embrace this journey with dedication and enthusiasm, and enjoy the positive impact it brings to your life.

THE END

www.ingramcontent.com/pod-product-compliance
Lightning Source LLC
Chambersburg PA
CBHW071841210526
45479CB00001B/240